BEING A DOCTOR

BEING A DOCTOR

THE ART OF MEDICINE

JOEL H. GOLDSTEIN, MD FAAO FACS

Outskirts Press, Inc.
Denver, Colorado

Acknowledgements

My parents were instrumental in enabling me to achieve my goal of becoming a physician.

Philip Goldstein (1910-1997) was a gifted high school and college biology teacher, author and creator of science study aids. He was always involved with his children. He cared. He was an educator and he encouraged my education, which led to my becoming a physician.

Margaret Garber Goldstein (1912-1991) was a loving wife and partner. She was also a loving, caring and involved mother who strongly supported my passion to be a physician.

I am grateful for their unwavering confidence in me.

Many people were of great help to me during the writing of this book.

My children and their spouses – Michael Goldstein, M.D., Jennifer

Rapaport, Robert Goldstein, J.D., Mara Goldstein, Deborah Goldstein, J.D., and David Sosnovick, M.D. – reviewed the book and provided many useful suggestions. Several friends, including Richard Abrams, M.D., Lawrence Laycob, M.D., Philip Wolf, M.D., Angela Wolf, R.N., and Stuart Heller also reviewed the manuscript and offered ideas for improvements. Particular thanks to Bernard Karshmer, Ph.D. who also provided pertinent suggestions and whose computer skills and tireless help made this project possible.

Special thanks also to Diana Wilson, Ph.D., with whom I previously enjoyed collaborating on a potential manuscript about the future of medicine. Some of the ideas we discussed are incorporated in this book.

My wife Lanie provided moral support and accepted my spending a lot of writing time at the computer. Special thanks to her for also putting up with many years of long hours away from home through medical school, internship, and residency and weeks of hibernation while studying for my boards, all the while dealing with two young children.

During medical school, internship and residency, and after, our education is derived from many medical mentors: full-time faculty, residents, and private practitioners. A few stand out as being particularly special to me. I would like to thank the following physicians who made major impacts on my medical career and education: Robert Glaser, C. Henry Kempe, Herbert Rothenberg, Phillip Wolf, Robert Sullivan, Kenneth Gottesfeld, Stuart Gottesfeld, Alan Hull, Barry Frank, Franz J. Ingelfinger, Norman Levinsky, Burton Polansky, the 1966-1967 House staff of the 5th and 6th Medical services at Boston City Hospital, Phillip Ellis, Kenneth Hovland, Marvin Lubeck, William Jackson, James Cerasoli, Lemuel

Moorman, George Moo Young, Hirsh E. Barmatz, Michael Goldstein, Andrew Mallory, Benzion Bub and Robert Sargent.

I deeply appreciate everyone's input, teaching, support, and help. Thank you to all.

Dedication

This book is dedicated to Hyman Heller, M.D. (1907-1969).

Dr. Heller, a graduate of Brown University and Rush Medical College, was the ultimate example of the caring physician. He was a man of many talents: college football player, professional basketball player, loving family man, and excellent family physician. He devoted his life to his general practice in Webster, Massachusetts, caring for his many patients who were frequently his friends and neighbors. He was well known for his superb diagnostic skills. He was active in local hospital and community affairs and was highly involved in the Worcester County Medical Society. His effective voice was instrumental in the decision by the state legislature to locate the newly created University of Massachusetts School of Medicine in the city of Worcester, rather than in the western part of the state as had been entertained and expected by many.

Dr. Heller was proud to be a physician. He was beloved by his patients, his friends, and his family.

Preface

Why this book?

I have been in medicine for over forty years. During this time I have seen huge changes in the knowledge base which physicians have to assimilate, and dramatic technologic improvements. But one thing has not changed: the practice of medicine is still based on a one-to- one, person-to-person relationship between the doctor and the patient. Medical schools do a wonderful job providing the knowledge base, but are lacking in the teaching of human interactions – the way to take care of people as the whole person, not a disease or an isolated organ which happens to be part of a body. We should be physicians first, specialists second.

This concept is not new, although it appears to be neglected. Francis W. Peabody, M.D. discussed the need for humanism in medicine in his famous paper, "The Care of the Patient," (JAMA 1927; 88:877-882), an essay which should be read by every medical practitioner.

Over the years I have developed my own way of taking care of patients which works well for my practice. I have distilled the ideas that have worked for me and have put them together into a presentation originally targeted to medical students and physicians in training, "The Art of Medicine." It has been suggested by others that this information might be of interest to a wider medical community, and I have therefore expanded on these thoughts and incorporated them into Parts I, II, and III of this book.

I have also added a fourth part which I thought might be helpful to those physicians finishing their training and about to enter the real world.

The fifth section includes some thoughts on, and hopes for, the future of medicine in the United States.

One cannot spend a lifetime in medicine without experiencing unusual situations and interesting people. Some are funny, some are sad. Some are frustrating, and some make you happy. I have included many such experiences in the body of the text, describing interesting, amusing, and unusual patient contacts which have occurred during my career. The medical vignettes scattered throughout the book are all based on actual patient encounters either in my practice or as experienced by other physicians.

Although I am an ophthalmologist, the information is this book is directed to all doctors in all areas of medicine. We are all physicians first!

It is my sincere hope that the information which follows will be of both interest and help to a variety of physicians at all levels, especially new physicians and those in training, and will provide topics for stimulating and thoughtful discussion.

Joel H. Goldstein, M.D.
Denver, Colorado, January 2011

Introduction

It is a joy to be a physician.

I am a doctor. I love what I do.

There is no occupation that provides greater satisfaction, intellectual stimulation, continuous learning, respect from the community, interpersonal relations, and the ability to help others. We are members of a privileged culture. We are privy to people's innermost secrets and fears. Patients divulge things to us they will tell no one else, even their closest friends or relatives. We are trusted more than any others, and as such we have a duty to be private in our conversations relating to what we have been told.

Our training is long, rigorous, intense, and expensive. We have sacrificed much to earn the title of medical doctor. It is truly an honor to be part of the culture of medicine. It requires great passion, dedication, commitment, and hard work. It also requires that we enjoy people, and want to be of service to them. We have to like to talk with people, share their happiness and their sad moments, and support their needs. We are healers, and as such enjoy our ability to help patients both emotionally and physically. Patients' lives and hopes are in our hands.

We have the opportunity to learn from, to teach, and to mentor other physicians. We are role models for younger doctors. We learn from those who have come before us. We are honored to be able to pass on our wisdom and experience to those who come after us.

It behooves us to be the most honest and ethical members of our society. We have great influence on our patients' attitudes and choices. We have the ability to convince patients based on our recommendations, to take or not take certain medicines, to accept or not accept certain treatments, to have or not have certain tests, and to have or not have a surgical procedure. We must not abuse this trust.

We are members of a unique fraternity of men and women and are lucky to be so. We have a special camaraderie with fellow doctors. We are happy in our choice of being physicians. It is fun to get up in the morning knowing you will face new challenges, meet new people, learn new things, and be of help to so many patients. I personally can think of nothing else I would rather be than a physician!

Table of Contents

Part I

To Be a Doctor

1

Overview-1

I am a Doctor!

After medical school I undertook a medical internship, spent two years as a general medical officer in the United States Air Force, and completed my ophthalmology residency in 1972. I have been in the private practice of ophthalmology in Denver, Colorado since that time.

You will be entering a whole new and different world.

During the many years since residency I have seen amazing changes in the practice of medicine: technically, socially, and culturally.

In my specialty, technological changes have included the operating microscope, phacoemulsification, intraocular lens implants, ocular coherence tomography, laser refractive surgery, and vastly improved cornea, intravitreal, and retinal surgeries. In other specialties the list includes MRI, CT scans, ultrasound, organ transplant surgery, Mohs surgery, interventional cardiology, cardiac imaging and cardiac surgery, functional artificial joints, sophisticated radiation therapy, the gamma knife, small incision and endoscopic surgery, robot surgery, DNA and genetic studies, genomics, gene therapy, and stem cell therapy. In addition, we have seen the development of a huge number of new oncologic and therapeutic agents.

Computers and electronic medical records have changed the culture of medicine. The electronic age has the potential to significantly improve the practice of medicine but also to alter the personal nature of medicine.

A major change in the practice of medicine involves the intrusiveness of government and insurance companies. Rules and regulations from these entities control reimbursement, what kinds of procedures and tests may be performed, and what therapeutic agents may be prescribed. Physician-owned facilities such as clinical laboratories, x-ray units, and ambulatory surgery centers are carefully scrutinized. Relationships between doctors and pharmaceutical companies are constantly being evaluated. Coding rules, audits, and billing denials have become part of the business of medicine.

Patient attitudes have undergone a significant cultural shift. In my early years of practice, good results were appreciated by patients. Now they expect perfection, partly due to unreasonable expectations created by physician marketing. Good often isn't enough any more. Patients frequently refuse to accept responsibility for their actions, and are quick to blame others for their medical situations. They often look for excuses to sue doctors for even minor medical or surgical incidents.

Financial responsibility is another area of concern. In most areas of commerce payment is expected when a service is provided or goods are purchased. There is a direct relationship between the provider and the purchaser. Not so for medicine. Third party intermediaries – Medicare, Medicaid, and private insurance companies – are positioned between the physician and the patient, paying for the majority of medical services. This situation has a significant negative effect on the physician-patient relationship. Patients do not expect to pay directly for medical services and in fact often resent requests for payment from medical offices. We hear statements such as "my insurance will pay for that" or even worse, "you can't charge for that, my insurance doesn't cover it." Patients blame the physician for services provided which their insurance companies deny, even when the service is appropriate and necessary. They assume the physician is acting wrongfully in these situations. Further, even though patients receive explanation of benefit forms, they fail to recognize the huge deductions from charges taken by insurance companies when payments are made to their physicians. Cost control is also made more difficult when patients are not directly responsible for the expenses of their medical care.

The other cultural change concerns relations between doctors. In many cases friendly professional relationships have been replaced by serious competition, marketing, jousting (bad-mouthing other physicians), and patient stealing. This has especially been a problem since the FTC approved physician advertising.

The medical world you will be entering is significantly different from the humanistic personal environment which I was privileged to enter just a few decades ago. You will need to be prepared for more competition, more outside control by non-medical elements, more governmental rules, regulations, and intervention, and more insurance company infringement, together with less personal autonomy, less humanism, more electronic decision-making, and less opportunity to create personal interactions with your patients and fellow physicians.

2

Overview-2

You've made it through college, medical school, internship, residency, and fellowship. Congratulations. Now it's time to grow up and face the real world. Once you made the decision to become a physician you had only to decide what schools to attend, which field of medicine to enter, and where to take your training. In the meantime your non-medical friends have been out the marketplace making real world decisions. You are about ten years behind them in worldly experience.

Now it's time to learn how to be a doctor, as well as a member of the business community. You need to know how to open and run an office, and how to take care of patients. You are part scientist, part businessman, and above all, a healer. Now, in whatever specialty, you will be involved with people, patients, other doctors, hospital employees, your own employees, drug and equipment salespeople, lawyers, insurance company representatives, the government – but primarily patients. You are in a service business; the practice of medicine is customer service at all levels.

Most physicians lack a business and financial mindset. Our interest is in people and in patient care, not in running a business. However, a medical office is a business. Physicians need the right combination of advisors, managers, and staff to enable them to run the office properly, while we, the physicians, follow our passion and interest: taking care of patients.

Your medical education emphasizes the science of medicine, not the art of medicine. Some people have this art intuitively, others must learn it, some never do. To be a great doctor you must be able to relate to people. Medical schools teach you about disease, pathology, technology, medicine, and surgery, but few teach students about the human element, taking care of the person. An exception is a course developed by Dr. Philip Wolf, professor of Cardiology at the University of Colorado Health Sciences Center, where he and a group of like-minded physicians mentor junior students in the art of medicine, and how it interacts with the science of medicine. I hope humanistic patient care as described in this book will be helpful for both new and experienced physicians at different career levels.

Doctors all follow different practice paths. Some will go solo, some will join private groups of varying sizes, some will join HMO models, some will be employed by hospitals, some will go into academic medicine, and some will go into research. All will have different concerns and needs, but what follows should be helpful to everyone. You just have to pick and choose what applies to you.

Part II

The Art of Medicine:
Doctor to Patient

3

Communication

A patient from a foreign country came in for an exam. When I asked what he came for his response was, "I'm not going to tell you." When I asked how I could help him his response was, "That's for you to find out." When I asked if he had any eye problems his response was, "You're the doctor. You tell me." He was obnoxious to say the least, but I accepted his challenge, performed his exam, figured out his problem, and sent him out happy.

In this section we will discuss the art of being a doctor. In essence, we should all follow the Golden Rule, and treat others as we would like to be treated. This means patients and their family members, other physicians, office staff, and hospital staff, as well as the variety of people with whom we come into contact during our day. Every person should be treated with respect. The keys to quality medical care – assuming a competent physician to begin with – include availability, accessibility, and communication.

LISTEN TO AND TALK WITH YOUR PATIENTS!

We must be available and accessible. Patients call, we respond. Other physicians call, we respond. Doctors should work appropriate hours so as to be available for our patients. We need to provide phone service where we can be reached, and we must return patient phone calls in a reasonable time frame. This is especially true when the call is after hours, an emergency, or when you are covering for another physician. Emergencies should be seen promptly. If the emergency happens to be your own patient, see them rather then pass them on to the on-call doctor. Patients cannot understand why their own physician can't see them when he or she is in the office seeing other patients, and they resent being sent off to a strange doctor. I am a member of a large call group for emergency evening, vacation, and weekend calls. One physician covers the group for a week at a time. I would occasionally get a call from a doctor who was in his or her office, but was "too busy" to see his or her own patient. The patient would be told to see the on-call physician. I was always happy to see them, but was always amazed a doctor who was in the office would send their patient elsewhere for urgent care. Patients resented being shunted off to another doctor when they knew their physician was present in the office. When your beeper goes off, answer it promptly and return the call promptly. When you are on call, stay around. Don't plan a trip out of town or go too far from home base, and of course, stay in beeper range. Be sure to have a pleasant, efficient answering service.

Unfortunately there are those patients who tend to abuse the emergency system.

I received a call from a patient from another doctor's office on a Saturday describing symptoms which had been present for three days. He had been too busy to call his regular physician during normal office hours. His symptoms were of a non-emergent nature and I advised the patient to call his physician for an evaluation after the weekend. He said no — he wanted to be seen on Saturday or Sunday, as it was not convenient for him to come in during the week.

A patient of mine called on a Friday morning asking me to see a friend of his who had ocular symptoms for two or three days for which he wanted to be evaluated. I advised him I was in the office and would be happy to see him. He told me he could not come until the end of the day, after office hours, because he was working and after all, it was a time and money situation. I advised him if it was a true emergency to come in and then go back to work. He never came.

When in your office, provide reasonable hours. If this is a new practice, you might find out when most doctors in your area take off, and plan to be in the office on those days. When I began my practice I found most local ophthalmologists were off on Wednesdays. I specifically worked on that day each week, and acquired many new patients in that way. Return in-office phone calls — ideally right away if urgent, the same day if non-urgent. Be sure your front desk is trained to triage the calls. They should be able to recognize which calls the physician must take, which can go to the technician, the optometrist, the physician's assistant, the nurse practitioner, or other office professional. They need to identify which calls need immediate phone response, which patients should be scheduled that day, and who could wait until later. Every specialty has certain buzz words the staff needs to recognize.

Make every attempt to see patients in a timely fashion. Do not be late arriving at your office. Be on time for your first patient in the morning and the afternoon. If you start late on a regular basis, patients will assume this is routine for you and will be unhappy. Your schedule will also be thrown off, as being a few minutes behind early in the day snowballs into longer and longer delays as the day goes on. Be efficient without seeming to rush. Patients should feel that when they are with you they are your only concern. Minimize interruptions when with a patient. Do not accept phone calls in your exam room unless absolutely necessary. I reviewed a legal complaint by an angry patient who was losing his vision and while his ophthalmologist was doing the eye exam, the doctor kept being interrupted to take calls from his stockbroker! Even worse, the patient could hear the conversations. The patient ended up with a poor visual result, and contacted an attorney. Although the final result was bad, and the physician's bedside manner was horrendous, he provided the appropriate treatment and there was no malpractice.

One of patients' biggest complaints is to be kept waiting, especially with no information as to the cause of the delay. If there will be an extended wait, have a staff person advise the waiting patients so they have the option of staying or rescheduling. Patients consider their time to be as valuable as yours.

4

Patient Feelings

Be considerate of your patients' feelings. Don't embarrass them. Don't be condescending. Don't yell at them, no matter how frustrated you may be. It seems unnecessary even to suggest these things, but they happen even with experienced physicians.

During medical school I was in an exam room with five male medical students for a cardiology teaching session. The patient was a young woman, undressed from the waist up, covered with a sheet. The attending cardiologist walked in, literally ripped off the sheet, and announced that we were all going to listen to her heart. He made no attempt to introduce himself, to explain anything to the patient, or to apologize for his rude behavior. The patient was mortified; we were embarrassed and apologized profusely. We learned little about her heart, but a lot about inappropriate physician actions.

In another situation, when we were learning to do pelvic exams, we were handed cold speculums which were obviously uncomfortable for the patients. I asked the teaching resident if the speculums could be warmed. After some discussion it was agreed and the policy became standard in the gynecology clinic.

BEING A DOCTOR

I have become aware of some physicians who literally yell at their patients when there is lack of rapid cooperation during an exam. Over the years I have acquired a number of such patients who refuse to go back to those doctors.

You cannot live by the clock alone. Patients will have problems which require giving up your lunch hour, or staying late after hours to deal with unexpected patient emergencies. There have been many nights when I was ready to leave the office, only to get a call or page about a patient who needed to be seen right away. It has always been my policy to stay and see those patients rather than send them to the ER or to the on-call physician. Often your staff will stay with you, as my staff often does, to help cover the emergency. Patients appreciate your willingness to go the extra mile for them. Of course there will always be situations where patients abuse your kindness in offering to help them, such as the lady who called at ten o'clock on a Saturday night to tell me about a problem which began seven hours earlier, or the lady with an emergency on a holiday weekend who refused my offer to meet her because she was having a pedicure, or the lady who couldn't come in because she had a hair appointment when I offered to see her for her emergency. As she explained, "Hair appointments are very hard to get, but doctors have to see patients for emergencies." She was right.

5

Interest in Patients

I performed cataract surgery on an elderly man. The result was excellent; he saw 20/20 in each eye and was very happy. A few months later, his wife came in to ask me a favor: "Put his cataracts back in." She was unhappy he could now see dust on the counter tops, dirt on the floor, and wrinkles on her face. She was particularly concerned because, "He didn't know I had wrinkles." She was serious about her request, and was disappointed I could not reverse the surgery.

Show interest in your patients. It's all right to talk about their family, their children and grandchildren, their accomplishments, their job, their awards, and the like. Patients appreciate the personal touch. In my chart I have a special page where I note personal comments about my patients. This page is not part of the official record. I also save clippings from papers and magazines relating to patients, and send copies to them with a note. I keep a copy in the chart. This allows me to bring up personal topics the next time I see the patients. They're usually amazed. After outpatient surgery I would ask the nurse to take a Polaroid photo of me with the patient and family members, then give the photo to the patient. They love it, and years later often bring the photo in to remind me of that day. Another way to use the pictures would be to have a photo wall in your office, but that may turn out to be a HIPAA violation. My office also sends thank you notes to friends or relatives for referrals, thank you notes for gifts, and condolence cards to family members of recently deceased patients. I will also go to the funerals of long-standing patients who have died. The families are surprised and pleased to know I was there. Patients like to know you care.

When I see a patient I always greet them and introduce myself with a handshake. I address them as Mr., Mrs., or Dr., not by their first name, unless they are well known to me or very young. Whenever possible and appropriate, I try to make a nice comment about how they look, or their jewelry, or their family, or their accomplishments if known to me. I always look at my special page (as noted in the paragraph above) to remind me about something unique about them. Individual compliments and comments make the visit personal and make the patient feel welcome and cared for. When the exam is over I always ask if they have any questions, tell them when I would like to see them again, and thank them for coming. I shake hands again when they leave. Touch is very bonding.

Communication is key to a happy patient base and a successful practice. Listen to your patients, and talk to them. Pay attention to their body language. Good doctors often know what is going on just by listening and looking before even doing an exam or any lab studies. The best doctors order tests and lab work to confirm a diagnosis, not to establish the diagnosis.

6

Think Outside the Box

A patient of mine for many years, a usually healthy and robust man, came in for his eye checkup. He was weak, had difficulty walking, and had to helped into the exam chair. He could barely hold his head up. I was shocked by his appearance, having seen him earlier in the year in his usual good health. On questioning it turned out he had been ill for several months, and despite treatment by his physician was deteriorating rapidly. I canceled the exam, and called another physician who I thought would be appropriate for this situation. He saw the patient immediately, made a different diagnosis, and instituted different treatment to which the patient quickly responded. The patient is again healthy, robust, and back to living his normal life.

It is important to think outside the box. Never accept the obvious at first glance. The head of radiology when I was in medical school, Dr. Marvin Daves, was fond of showing students a chest X-ray with an obvious large lung tumor. Invariably the students would identify the tumor, but totally miss the more subtle abnormal area in another part of the lung. His point: ignore the obvious, look for and think of other possibilities, and identify the obvious last.

On the other hand, use common sense when making a diagnosis. Don't look for esoterica when you can make a reasonable diagnosis. The famous medical saying: "When you hear hoofbeats look for horses, not zebras," applies most of the time.

Remember no matter what your specialty, you are still a physician and must be alert to patient problems beyond their presenting symptoms or their supposed reason for coming to see you. I have had the opportunity to help many patients who came in for ophthalmic evaluation but had medical needs which were far more important their eye situation.

In my early years in practice, when cataract surgery was an in-hospital procedure and we did our own preoperative histories and physicals, I found a breast mass in a patient who was scheduled for cataract surgery the next day. She had been unaware of the lesion. I called a general surgeon, and canceled her cataract surgery. The mass was removed and was malignant. The patient did well. Her cataract was removed later after she recovered from her cancer therapy.

On two occasions, about a year apart, I came into my exam room to face an obviously anxious, distraught female patient. In both situations it turned out each woman had been diagnosed with a breast mass which required biopsy. The surgeons to whom they were referred were to perform the biopsy in three to four weeks' time. The patients were scared. I immediately called an excellent surgeon who I knew would understand the need for more rapid surgery. The women were seen and underwent biopsy within twenty-four hours. In each case the lesion was malignant. Both women were treated appropriately and have done well.

A long-standing patient came in for a glaucoma pressure test. He did not look his usual healthy self. On questioning it turned out he had had some chest pain and dyspnea for a week. I recommended he be seen immediately for a cardiac evaluation. He refused, saying he was all right. I then called his primary care physician, told him the story, and he advised the patient to come right over to his office. The patient did have a blocked coronary vessel which required a stent.

I saw a lady who although usually healthy, looked pale and ashen. I thought she had anemia and recommended she see her primary care physician immediately who found her to be significantly anemic. She is now on iron and is doing well.

A glaucoma patient who had been on a beta-blocker eye drop for a long time came in for an eye pressure check and was obviously having shortness of breath, which he had not had before. I referred him for a cardiac work-up. He turned out to have a blocked coronary vessel and required a stent.

7

Honesty

All doctors must be exceedingly honest. If you cannot see or hear the problem, say so! Do not make up what you cannot hear or see. My pediatrics chief in medical school, Dr. C. Henry Kempe, chastised several of my classmates when they described having seen the tympanic membrane, and the middle ear bones in an ear whose canal was filled with cerumen, obscuring the ear drum. His point: describe what you actually see, and never make up what you did not or cannot see. Dr. Phillip P. Ellis, long time chairman of ophthalmology at the University of Colorado Health Sciences Center, drummed into his residents the importance of honesty in the practice of medicine. Cardiology instructors enjoy asking students to describe heart sounds and murmurs which do not exist, to test their honesty.

8

Tests and Diagnosis

Early in my career, an elderly grandmother came in for an exam. I told her she was fine, and among other things she did not have glaucoma. Her response was, "Damm, I wanted glaucoma!" I was quite surprised, as most patients are happy not to have glaucoma. It turned out she liked marijuana brownies, and figured if she had glaucoma she could get the marijuana legally.

When you are with a patient, don't rush. Listen to them, think, do appropriate exams and tests, and tell them what is going on. Do not talk in medical language. Remember, the terms we take for granted often sound like a foreign language to our patients. This is especially true in certain specialties such as ophthalmology. Do not talk down to patients. Use common words which would generally be understood by most non-medical people. Do not be condescending, or you may never see that patient again. Don't rush out the door, but learn how to end a conversation. Patients really don't want you to leave once they have you in the room. Make them feel important, but don't let them monopolize your time. You do have others waiting.

BEING A DOCTOR

Doctors order tests. Patients are anxious to know the results. Every doctor's office must follow up on all test results and inform the patients as to the findings. Physicians must review all test results, sign off on them, and be sure either they or their staff advise the patient as to the results. The test and the information relayed to the patient should be documented in the chart. It is also important to document attempts to contact the patient as they often complain later that no one tried to reach them when in fact they ignored or didn't pick up messages. Normal test results can be relayed to the patient by staff members. The physician should discuss abnormal tests with the patient directly, either by phone or in person, depending on the significance of the test. Patients often incorrectly assume no call from the doctor's office means the test is normal, or at least not worrisome. Patients should be instructed to call if they don't learn about a test result within a reasonable time interval, say a week.

Once you have made your diagnosis, explain. Discuss treatment, expectations, need for surgery where indicated, and prognosis. When possible, and if appropriate, involve family members. Patients will not remember a great deal of what you say, especially if you are talking about a significant problem. It helps to have another pair of ears in the room, and most of the time family members want and need to know also. If surgery is recommended, be sure to explain the benefits, potential risks, and what the patient may expect to go through before, during, and after the procedure. Patients especially need to be informed about what to expect after surgery, restrictions, activities, return to work, medications, frequency of follow-up visits, what problems to look for, and when it might be appropriate for them to call the office. Don't forget, what we take for granted is all new to the patient. You may have done a procedure many times, but for the patient this is probably the first time. Never be blasé about surgery! Be complete with your informed consent. Where possible, do it yourself. I personally go over the informed consent with all my refractive surgery patients, and answer their questions myself.

If you notice an unusual finding which you know to be insignificant, or congenital with no consequences, tell the patient anyway. We live in a mobile society; the patient might see another doctor elsewhere who may mention the finding to an incredulous patient who knew nothing about it. The second physician may consider it something new, which might require unnecessary testing.

If you don't know the answer, that's okay. Patients appreciate honesty. Be comfortable requesting an opinion from another physician, or referring the patient out. No one knows everything, especially in medicine. No one is best at every operation. In general, do what you are good at and let others do what they do well. You need to be the best you can be. Patients appreciate that philosophy. Do not try to be all things to all people.

If a patient does have surgery, be sure to communicate with the waiting family. They will be anxious, and will want to hear from you as soon as is reasonable. Do not prolong the time before you talk with them, even if the case is short. I have heard of physicians who sit in the doctors' surgical lounge after surgery, making the family wait, so they will think the procedure was longer than it really was. This is wrong. Family members are nervous. When you're done, go talk to them. If the case is running later than expected, send word out to the family to explain. Give good written post-operative instructions so the family knows what to do and what to expect. I once worked with a surgeon who, when he met with the family after surgery, would hand them medicine with the statement, "Here's a tube of ointment not to use." He would then turn away and return to the operating suite, leaving very confused relatives in his wake. I had to explain that the tube was given just in case it was needed later. This is clearly not the way to talk to the family when a loved one has just had a surgical procedure.

After outpatient surgery it's a nice touch to call patients at home the night of surgery to see how they are doing. You'll be amazed at the surprise in their voice – "I can't believe you're calling me," – and at how pleased they are to hear from you. This phone call may also save you a wake-up call in the middle of the night. It is generally a good idea to see your patient on the day after surgery for a post-operative check, depending on the type of surgery done. It's also a good time to remind them and their family about the post-op medicine regime.

9

Complications

Over the years I have reviewed many cases for attorneys to evaluate potential malpractice. The vast majority were complications, but not malpractice, and I have been able to avert many lawsuits for many physicians. In one situation, which was malpractice, I asked the plaintiff attorney if I could meet with the defense attorney to see if I could convince the defense to settle the case without a trial. He demurred, saying, "That's not how we do things." A few weeks later he called to tell me the defense was wiling to meet. We did, the case was settled shortly after our meeting, and the physician was spared the agony of a long drawn-out malpractice case.

Do not walk away from complications. Doctors tend to have big egos, and do not like to admit to mistakes, failures, or bad results. If there is a problem, patients need extra support. They want you to tell them what happened, why – if you know – and what you are going to do to help them get through the situation. You must be there for them. Be honest. Apologize when appropriate. Patients do not want to feel abandoned by their physicians. Over the years I have reviewed many potential malpractice cases for attorneys. The vast majority were not malpractice, but situations where the result was not good, and the physician essentially backed off from explaining things to the patient and accepting responsibility. Even worse, in many cases the physician actually avoided dealing with the patient, leaving the patient to feel abandoned by their physician. Essentially the physician was not there for the patient. It's easy for them to then start thinking about malpractice. Although most of these potential suits can be prevented by an honest review by an outside physician, they should never have been instigated in the first place.

Talk to your patients. Be there for them. Respect them.

10

First Do No Harm

I saw a patient who was essentially blind from cataracts. He literally could not see the hand in front of his face. He told a sad story. About four years prior to his visit to me he was a commercial truck driver with excellent vision. He started to develop cataracts, and went to a "doctor" who prescribed eye drops which he sold to the patient with the understanding they were designed to prevent the growth of cataracts. The patient purchased and used the drops faithfully, visited the "doctor" frequently for years and was told each time he was doing well with no cataract growth. His vision continued to deteriorate to the point he could not see well enough to drive, and lost his job. He continued to believe the "doctor." He finally got to the visual level where he was unable to care for himself due to his poor vision. A neighbor brought him to my office where I found cataracts so dense it was impossible to examine the inside of his eye. I performed cataract surgery, his vision returned to 20/20, and he regained his job. He threw the drops away!

Primum non nocere. "First, do no harm."

We must consider the consequences of our actions. We must balance risk and benefit for each service we provide for our patients and make our interventional decisions accordingly. Even in the best of circumstances, mistakes will occur, and decisions will be made which may result in complications. However, whatever action we take must be made in the best interests of our patients. We should not provide services for our patients which are either wrong or inappropriate, especially if done for financial gain.

We all have seen complications occur from surgical procedures or medical decisions when inadvertent damage may be done to one structure or organ while trying to save or fix another. Such potential risks are usually known and should be explained to patients beforehand.

Such is not the case when poor judgment or judgment based on financial remuneration causes physicians to provide inappropriate services.

One of the original refractive eye procedures was radial keratotomy. For patients who wore hard contact lenses, which distort the cornea, it was necessary for them to stay out of lenses for months to allow corneal shape normalization before having surgery.

I saw a patient who had radial keratotomy done on one eye after being out of hard lenses for only a week. The surgery further distorted her already distorted cornea, resulting in poor vision. After weeks of patient complaints, the surgeon foolishly redid the operation, making the vision worse. After several more weeks when the vision failed to improve, the surgeon suggested doing the second eye, "in the meantime", even though the first eye continued to demonstrate poor visual recovery. At this point the patient came to me for a second opinion. I recommended no further surgery be done. After several months of healing, we were able to refit the first eye with a new contact lens which provided functional vision. This patient was harmed inappropriately by this surgery and received no benefit.

I evaluated a patient for laser refractive surgery who had thin corneas and a highly myopic prescription. I advised against surgery as this combination of findings could be expected to result in an unstable cornea. She went elsewhere, found a surgeon to do her LASIK procedure, and ended up with unstable fluctuating vision. Since a hard contact lens did not help, she will probably need a corneal transplant to stabilize her vision. This patient should never have had surgery in the first place.

I opened my first office in the Cherry Creek area of Denver. I was unaware that an optometrist with the same last name had an established practice in Cherry Creek less than a mile from my office. I quickly learned how often patients confuse optometrists with ophthalmologists. A number of patients who had been referred to me by other patients and doctors mistakenly went to him. He acted as though he knew the referring person and took care of the patients as if they had been referred to him. I learned of the situation later, when the patients came to me the next time after learning of their error. The only time he would advise them they were in the wrong place was when they either had Medicaid, or no insurance. In one instance a tragedy was averted. He had told a patient she had a retina problem which was not amenable to treatment; nothing could be done to help her. Had she taken his word, she would have lost significant vision. Luckily, being scared by this news, she called her referring internist who, realizing she went to the wrong doctor, called me. The patient turned out to have a problem amenable to laser therapy which was performed. The patient did well; her vision was saved. After five years in this location, I moved to another office in a different area of Denver and the problem with this optometrist eventually ended.

Part III

The Art of Medicine: Doctor to Doctor

11

Accessibility and Communication

An attractive lady came in for an eye exam dressed as though she was going to a fancy party. When I asked why she was dressed in such an elaborate way she explained, "After I finish here I'm going to see my pediatrician." When I acted surprised, she said, "All the ladies get dressed up when they go to see him." It turned out the pediatrician was a friend and classmate of mine, a man who was totally professional. I knew he would be embarrassed had he known his patients' mothers would get all dressed up for him. In fact he and his partner, also a classmate, were the pediatricians for my own children.

It is vitally important to be available and accessible to other physicians. Ideally, a person, not a machine, should answer the phone in your office. Neither patients nor physicians like a phone menu, and the more options it has, the more likely one is to hang up. You should have a special line for doctors. If you must have a phone menu, make option number one your physician line. No doctor will tolerate waiting through several voice prompts to get to the one that says, "If you are a doctor or doctor's office, push this number." When you do get a physician call, stop, if possible, and take it immediately. Remember, he or she is just as busy as you are. They may be calling to send you a patient, or a consult, or an emergency, all of which are essential to your practice development. This is even more important if you are a specialist, or are just opening a practice. You need to be available if you expect to get referrals. Be gracious. Be happy to receive another physician's overflow, consults, and requests for help or advice. Thank them. Doctors like to refer patients to doctors who are receptive. The reverse is also true. No one likes to feel as though you think you are doing them a favor by taking their patients. They are actually doing you a favor by sending patients to your office. Referrals dry up quickly if you are not happy to accept them.

During my first year in practice I enjoyed many fully scheduled days thanks to the kindness of several local ophthalmologists, especially Dr. Marvin Lubeck and Dr. William Jackson, who frequently referred their overflow patients to me in order to help me establish my practice.

Traditional medical teaching is based on a mentoring system. Experienced physicians teach those who follow in their footsteps. Professors, residents, and fellows teach students. Junior doctors in training are taught by those more senior, and doctors in practice teach younger doctors with whom they come in contact. Doctors in practice also learn from other physicians with whom they share patients. There is a general sharing of knowledge and experience. Such teaching should be positive, as has been demonstrated for years by Dr. Kenneth Hovland, a retina specialist in Denver, who has been instrumental in educating residents, fellows, private ophthalmologists, and eye care professionals around the world where he travelled on the ship *Hope* and with Project Orbis. An example of the opposite, negative teaching, would be a chief resident in surgery with whom I came in contact during medical school and whose policy was to be condescending to students and residents, and to educate by fear. As a result, no student wanted to scrub in surgery when he was operating, and the junior residents over whom he was in charge were intimidated and afraid. As you might expect, my medical school class had a very low percentage of students who chose general surgery for their career. The chief of surgery was concerned, but chose to interview only those few students who were committed to surgical residencies. As a result he learned nothing of the true situation, and no changes were made.

Communication with other physicians is critical to your success. Remember that the terminology for your specialty may be foreign to their ears. For example, ophthalmology has a language of its own and is unintelligible to most physicians. When I did my medical internship and requested ophthalmology consults, we had no idea what was being said; it was all written in ophthalmology abbreviations! As a result of that experience, I am careful to respond to consultations requests in clear English, in medical terms understood by non-ophthalmic physicians.

Communication with physicians and other health care providers is also important on another level relating to patient care. Poor communication can affect patient safety and create liability. Failure to communicate between health care providers can lead to consequences for the patient. When signing off on care from one doctor to another, be sure the accepting physician knows all about the patient: diagnosis, tests performed, medications ordered, and special needs. The same is true when a patient is transferred from an emergency room physician to another physician. When in surgery, nurses and surgeons must communicate about the surgery to be done. The nurse and the surgeon must discuss which body part requires surgery, and be sure the correct area is being prepped. There have been cases reported of the wrong extremity being prepped. When the surgeon entered the room, all he or she saw was a draped extremity ready for surgery, operated assuming it was the correct extremity, only to find out after surgery that it was not. The number of wrong patient, wrong extremity, or wrong organ operations should be zero. Unfortunately such is not the case. Surgeons must be diligent in assuring the correct operation is performed on the correct part of the body of the correct patient. Proper communication in the operating room is essential.

The book Waking up Blind *by Tom Harbin, M.D., describes a case at a major medical center where a patient was to have surgery on his abnormal right eye, but instead underwent surgery on his essentially normal left eye, resulting in significant visual loss to the patient.*

I have treated a patient who underwent refractive eye surgery by another physician where a different patient's prescription was mistakenly placed in the computer, resulting in a poor visual outcome.

When doctors call, respond. Take their calls, respond to their messages, see their consults, and accept their overflow. When you do see a patient, send a report promptly. Sometimes it is better to call first, and send the report later.

If the emergency room doctor calls, take the call. He or she needs your help and support. See the patient if necessary, or explain to him or her how to take care of the problem. In certain specialties, such as ophthalmology, it is useful to spend some time with the ER team explaining the use of the slit lamp and the basics of eye care. These few hours can save you many late night calls. Of course, the ER is also a good source of new patients for the beginning physician.

12

Consultation

Most patients are pleasant and appreciative, but during a long career every physician encounters patients who are difficult, even obnoxious. Luckily they are few and far between. During my first year in practice I was referred an elderly lady who — little did I know at the time — would turn out to be the most unpleasant patient I have ever seen in my entire career. Her referring physician apologized before she even came to my office, advising she was the most difficult patient he had ever taken care of in his many years of practice, but he thought I would be up to the challenge. She was in fact exceedingly difficult, demanding, unappreciative, and entitled. I soon found out that she had been dismissed from the practices of almost every physician who had ever cared for her, including one practice where the police were called to remove her from the doctor's office when she arrived without an appointment, caused a stir in the waiting room, and would not leave voluntarily. I also found that even though she was exceedingly wealthy, she would not pay any bills until threatened with collections. About two weeks after her first appointment with me, I received a box containing a dozen long- stemmed roses. The note inside said, "Dear Joel, it is a pleasure to have friends like you." It was signed by her previous ophthalmologist!

When referring patients to other physicians for opinions or

consultations, call the physician ahead of time to prepare him or her for the patient's arrival. Send them whatever tests you have done which might be helpful. It is inappropriate for you to send the patient with no advance information. I know of situations where a physician would find a patient in his waiting room with serious problems and no records or information relating to the case. "Dr. X told me to show up here." Often the patient cannot explain his or her situation, and the referring doctor may have been too embarrassed to call the consultant because of the poor quality of his or her care, or just from lack of courtesy or consideration for the specialist.

It would be a good idea to develop a network of quality physicians you trust and respect to whom you can refer patients, knowing they will be properly cared for and that you will receive appropriate evaluations.

When you receive a consult, be careful to provide the information or care requested. There are basically two types of consult: one where you are asked for an opinion and recommendations, the other where you are requested to assume care of the patient. It's nice to call the referring doctor, but always provide a written report promptly. It's embarrassing for the requesting physician to see the patient after the consult, and have no information as to what was diagnosed or recommended. Do not provide extra services unless requested or necessary. I used to refer patients for consults to a local glaucoma specialist, but found that in addition to taking care of the glaucoma, he would remove their cataracts. I stopped referring to his office.

If you think the referring physician missed something important, or

CONSULTATION

if you find something of concern which might require referral to a different specialist, call and discuss the situation with the physician who referred the patient to you. Don't take it on yourself to make a new referral without the concurrence of the original physician. There are situations where the consultant takes over the patient and then refers within their own circle of friends, some of whom may not be acceptable to the original referring physician. This is a sure way of guaranteeing the loss of future referrals from that physician.

However, there may be extenuating circumstances where recommending a new referral without consultation with the original physician may be appropriate.

13

Personal Relationships

Personal relations with other physicians are of great importance. If you are joining a group, be supportive of your partners, especially with regard to patient care. If you disagree with the philosophy of your partner, discuss it with him or her, not with the patient. If you are an older physician who takes in a younger partner, be especially supportive and do not be jealous if the new partner does well and develops a practice of his or her own, which may eventually be more successful than yours. You should be pleased and proud that you selected a good young doctor to work with you. In my community I have seen both situations. In one case a senior doctor called me one day to tell me how happy he was that in just a few years his new younger associate was already bringing in more practice income than he was. Their association lasted for about forty years before the senior physician's retirement. The opposite occurred in another office where the senior man brought in excellent younger physicians who would be fired when they started to do well on their own.

14

Jousting

During my early years in practice I took care of a law student from a local university. He was very demanding, but since I was new in practice I tried to accommodate his needs, scheduling his numerous appointments to coincide with his school schedule. He seemed happy with my services, but when it came to paying, he forgot about all the efforts I made in his behalf. He sent a check for a fraction of the bill, marked "paid in full," together with a letter written on stationery from a law firm where he was clerking, threatening a malpractice suit if I didn't cancel the rest of the bill. I considered sending a copy of his inappropriate letter to the dean of the law school, but after discussion with attorney friends of mine, I decided not to as it might have been detrimental to the student's career. I never cashed the check.

It is wrong for physicians to denigrate other physicians in the presence of patients. This is known as jousting. It can lead to unhappy patients and malpractice suits. I know of a case where a patient underwent surgery with a good result, but the patient felt it should have been better. He self-referred to a specialist who advised him the surgery was fine and needed more healing time. He then went to another doctor who, in an unnecessary attempt to improve the outcome, did a procedure which actually made the patient worse and subsequently required several more surgeries by yet another doctor to repair. This physician then told the patient the problem was the fault of the original physician, not him, even though he caused the damage. His negative comments about the work of the original surgeon caused the patient to file a malpractice suit against that surgeon. After two years of legal discourse and meetings, many depositions, and a great deal of time and expense, the suit was eventually withdrawn before trial. Had it not been for jousting, It would never have been filed in the first place.

Other forms of jousting include the doctor who told a patient he met at a party to leave his present physician and come to him because he would do a better job taking care of the patient's medical situation. The patient chose to stay with his original physician. Or the doctor who saw a patient for another physician in an emergency situation. He treated the emergency and in addition, advised the patient that the medical treatment for her unrelated chronic condition was not adequate and that she needed surgery for which she should come to him. The patient reported back to her original doctor who continued her appropriate medical treatment and advised her surgery was not necessary. The patient has continued to do well without surgery for over thirty years.

Doctors should not tell attorneys that bad results are malpractice if they are not, just to get paid to review a case. In some states a physician must agree there is potential malpractice before a case can be filed. For example, Colorado requires a certificate of review by a qualified doctor. Physicians should not make such a statement just for money, but should honestly feel there may be malpractice before authorizing a case to be filed. I was an expert witness for the defense in a malpractice case in which there was clearly no malpractice, but where the plaintiff attorney found a physician in another state who, for a large fee, was willing to provide the necessary certificate of review to authorize that a case for malpractice be filed. The defense won after several years of wasted time and expense. Doctors are wrong to act in this way. We should not testify or report against other physicians for the money when there is no malpractice. Don't be too quick to judge too harshly. Remember the saying about people in glass houses. Going through a malpractice case as a defendant is painful, emotionally destructive, expensive, and time-consuming. On the other hand, we do have an obligation to be honest in situations which we truly believe to be malpractice.

Physicians also should not create an excuse to call an action malpractice in order to justify their participation as an expert witness. I was a defense expert in a case which involved two different questions of standard of care where a physician did two separate procedures on the same patient. The plaintiff expert advised there was malpractice involving one procedure. He could not find failure of the standard of care in the second procedure, so he essentially said that because he felt the defendant physician was negligent in the first procedure, he therefore must have been negligent during the second procedure also. This is obviously an absurd position.

Over the years I have reviewed many potential malpractice cases for attorneys. Most of these complaints were not malpractice, and I have been able to advise the plaintiff attorneys not to file these cases. The vast majority were based on complaints by unhappy patients who may have had bad results, but were really angry because their doctors blew them off by refusing to answer questions, not being available, or demonstrating poor bedside manner. Essentially, the physician was not there for the patient. We must bend over backwards to be supportive to our patients in situations where there are poor outcomes, no matter what the cause. We physicians must accept responsibility for our actions and our results. The buck stops with us!

It is important to support community physicians. Do not bad-mouth other physicians. It serves only to make you look small. It might even make patients think about the idea of a malpractice suit. It is better to say nice things about other doctors, assuming they are true. It makes the patient feel good about their previous physician, and makes you look like a bigger person. I always compliment other doctors' work when I can honestly do so. Patients appreciate knowing they have chosen appropriate physicians.

15

Hospitals and Nurses

Get involved in your hospital. Be active on the staff. Join committees and become active in administrative activities. You will learn a lot about the medical environment, will quickly get to know your fellow physicians, and will meet a lot of non-physicians who care about health care. You will also get referrals. Take ER calls, especially if you are a new physician. You will make many contacts, and increase your business.

Nurses are important people. They are professionals. Treat them with respect. Utilize their abilities. Do not be condescending. This is especially true in surgery, where I have seen nurses verbally abused by surgeons who appear to handle stress by mistreating all those around them. There is never an excuse to yell at your operating room support team, or to throw surgical instruments. Treat nurses well. They will make your life easier in all aspects of patient care, and will take better care of your patients. Physicians and nurses are on the same team, and have the same goal: to provide excellent compassionate care for the patient. Nurses will also be a good source of referrals. Nurses are happy to send patients to those doctors who treat them nicely, and who they feel provide excellent patient care. It is interesting to see how often the two go together. Doctors who are nice to nurses and other support staff tend to be nicer to and take better care of their patients also.

Part IV

Going into Practice

16

Joining a Practice

While preparing for the opening of my office, phone calls were call forwarded to my home number. A lady called stating she had seen me before and wanted to be my very first patient in my new office. I was of course very excited and put her as number one in my brand new appointment book. The big day arrived, my first day in practice. In walked the lady. I came out to greet her with great anticipation. She looked at me and said, "Who are you? I'm looking for Dr. Goldstein." When I explained that's who I was she said, "You're not the Dr. Goldstein I was looking for. I've never seen you before." Needless to say I was disappointed, but she stayed for an exam anyway and remained my patient for many years.

The basics of opening or joining a practice include many facets.

You will need legal counsel in a variety of specialties. Your lawyers must know about business – especially contracts, liability, employment, estate planning, health care law, tax, and malpractice. You might be best served by a multi-specialty firm which provides a variety of expertise, or you may rely on individual attorneys on an as- needed basis.

BEING A DOCTOR

You will need a good CPA, preferably one who is experienced in medical accounting matters.

You will need to embrace many types of insurance. Life insurance, whole or term, is to be considered for you and possibly your spouse and your family. Health insurance for you, your family, and your employees will be very important, especially in deciding how much will be paid for and by whom. Disability – hopefully based on your specific abilities and specialty, rather than providing general coverage as a physician – is important, but more difficult to purchase than in the past. Malpractice coverage from a reputable carrier is a must. Remember to get enough coverage. Don't skimp, and don't forget the need for tail coverage after you leave practice. Ideally, you want a carrier which is not quick to settle inappropriate claims, and gives you the option of refusing to settle a claim, or at least considers your opinion in regard to settlement. You should consider long-term insurance, realizing the younger you start, the cheaper the premiums. From an office standpoint you will need worker's comprehensive insurance, and office equipment protection, together with insurance for staff salaries, your own salary, and office overhead expenses, in case you are unable to practice for a time.

If you are buying into a practice a retinue of advisors will be needed, including an attorney specializing in contracts, a CPA, and a medical office practice appraiser. You want to be sure you will be compatible with the physicians already in the practice. You need to understand the terms of remuneration for you and other practice members, bonus plans, expected work hours and patient load, on-call demands, days off schedules, vacation times, buy-in requirements, partnership arrangements, retirement plans, and retirement strategies for senior partners. It is easy for the existing members of the group to take advantage of the new member in terms of work load expectations, time off, and remuneration. Everything possible should be spelled out in writing. Be especially careful if family members of the partners hold important positions in the office. I know of at least one office where the physician's spouse was the office manager, and newly recruited physicians were kept totally in the dark with regard to office finances. They usually left after a short time, feeling taken advantage of, often with bitter feelings. Talk to as many doctors as you can who have entered into similar situations, especially those who might have been in the same practice you are looking at and may no longer be there. What did they like, and what did they dislike? What did they do right and what did they do wrong? If not there any more, why did they leave? You should also be fair in your expectations with regard to work load, hours, vacations, and remuneration. Your new practice situation should be based on a win-win arrangement, and should not be one sided in either direction.

Coding knowledge is crucial to your financial success. You should personally take coding courses in your specialty, and should ideally have a coding professional working in your office. This is feasible in a larger practice, but may be more difficult financially in a small office. The more you have to do yourself, the more you need to be educated. Your income depends on correct coding! Insurance evaluators are quick to down code (down coding has become an industry unto itself), but you can be sure they will not advise when you have coded lower than you should.

If you are opening your own office, you will need help with space planning and office interior design. You want to be sure your office layout is efficient, demonstrates little wasted space, allows for privacy, and works for your needs — those of your staff, and especially those of your patients. Be sure your office is attractive, comfortable, and presents a pleasant environment for work and for your patients.

17

Human Resources

The most obscure area for doctors to relate to may be human resources. Hiring and firing employees is not part of what we have been trained to do. It is not easy to evaluate potential employees. Be sure job applicants are screened carefully. Check references. Test abilities to perform necessary tasks. Evaluate personality for compatibility; do not accept stated qualifications at face value. Meet and interview candidates. Have a ninety-day probation period, with the ability to fire without cause during this time. It will also be difficult for the physicians to supervise employee job performance and, if necessary, to fire them. States differ in their rules and regulations with regard to hiring and firing, but in general the pendulum leans toward the employee, not the employer. It can be very difficult and expensive to remove someone from your office, even with cause. If you are joining a larger organization you should hope they have a qualified human resources person on board. If you are solo or in a small practice, this may be a big challenge. You will definitely need a competent office manager or human resource person to monitor employees.

BEING A DOCTOR

I once hired an employee who I later found out lied about her work experience and her abilities. She also brought her teenage son to help her do computer work, with which she had claimed to be proficient, but was not. I allowed him to work during the day and paid him, as she was a single mom and I felt sorry about her situation, trying to help her financially in this way. After a time I learned she was bringing him in to work after hours, when the staff and I had gone home. I advised her this was inappropriate and illegal, and requested she stop this activity. It was not long before it became obvious she was unable to perform her duties for a job she had lied to get. I fired her. The next thing I knew she filed a complaint with the state labor board, and as part of her complaint she accused me of child labor abuse, based on the fact that her son was working after hours, which I specifically had told her he should not do! She also named another employee in the complaint, without either her knowledge or consent. I called the labor board to explain the dishonesty of the complaint. I was told they were not interested in the employer's side of the story, and that their responsibility was to support the employee. I was forced to hire an attorney at significant expense, while her costs were absorbed by the state. I won.

I also learned some good lessons. Check references. Test potential employee proficiency. Document every infraction by your employees, no matter how minor. Don't expect any help from your state. Their interest is with employees, not employers.

The list of job descriptions for a medical office can be long, depending on the size of your office and your budget. If you are joining an established organization, it is likely that these people will already be in place. The disadvantage is you may have little say in hiring and firing, even if your experience with a particular employee may not be positive. This is especially true in a more bureaucratic organization such as a medical school or a large multi-specialty practice. If you are starting out, you will need to think about an office manager, a human resources person (who could also be the office manager), and front desk people to answer phones, check patients in and out, collect money and super-bills, and monitor the waiting room. In ophthalmology you also may need optometrists and/or ophthalmic technicians to help with patient care. Other specialties may require other professional ancillary help such as nurses, physician assistants, nurse midwives, or child health associates.

Billing is, of course, the lifeblood of your office. You will need to decide whether to keep billing in-house, or to outsource it. Keeping it in-house gives you better control, while outsourcing gives you continuity and possibly more accuracy. You need someone who understands insurance, how to respond to contracts, and how to deal with insurance company demands and payment denials. Many smaller offices depend on outside professionals for this. Depending on office size, you may need a medial records coordinator. If you do a lot of specialized work, such as an ophthalmologist who does LASIK, you may require a LASIK coordinator. Transcription is another area which could be in-house, or outsourced. You may need a coding specialist.

18

Employees

During internship I was wheeling a patient on a gurney through the basement tunnels connecting the Boston City Hospital buildings from the emergency room to the ward. My ward was on the fifth floor. The elevators in the buildings were not self-service. Rather, they were manned by Boston city employees. When I finally got to the elevator door in the basement of our building, I rang the buzzer. No response. This went on for about fifteen minutes, continuous ringing with no response. I asked a passing nurse to watch the patient, and sprinted up the stairs until I found the upper floor where the elevator was parked. The operator was having a fine time drinking coffee with the ward nurses, ignoring the elevator bell. I commandeered the elevator, took it down to the basement, brought my patient to the floor, then deposited the elevator in the basement and left it there with the door open so the operator was forced to climb down the stairs to retrieve it. I could hear his voice cursing in the stairwell as he went down when he realized his elevator was missing.

Treat your employees with respect. Hire good people, train them, and keep them. Check references. Give raises as deserved. I know a physician who would fire good employees when they became eligible for a raise. He was penny wise and pound foolish.

Encourage independent thinking and action. Make them feel valued as members of the office team. You want your employees to feel invested in the success of your office. Don't micromanage. Hire a good manager. Reward good work. Be supportive. Give praise for good work. People like to be recognized. Never criticize in front of other employees or patients. Be sure they understand your expectations and their job description. Encourage teamwork. Give small tokens of appreciation (money, gift certificates, movie passes, restaurant certificates, tickets to ball games or theater) for especially good work. Base a bonus system on meeting productivity goals.

Employees must recognize that they represent you. They must look and act professional. They must be welcoming, look up and make eye contact with patients. They must acknowledge the patient's arrival. They must be pleasant, happy, neat and clean, and present a nice appearance. They need to recognize patients on arrival and ensure an efficient check-in. They must be pleasant on the phone. They need to be able to handle difficult patients in person and on the phone. They should call patients by their last names, especially older people. They must respect the privacy of every patient.

They should not eat at the front desk, talk on personal cell phones, text message, use the computer for personal matters, or gossip within earshot of patients. They should not talk loudly at the front desk so patients in the waiting room can hear, especially when talking to other patients on the phone.

19

Electronic Medical Records

Computerized medical records have great potential to improve the practice of medicine. They also have the potential to detract from personal care, and they will open up new avenues for legal attacks on the medical profession. Electronic medical records must be designed and used carefully and thoughtfully. Security and protection of patient information will be a major area of concern and must be addressed at all levels.

Like it or not, electronic medical records will be required due to federal mandates. This is a problem for established practices, due to expense, training, integration of existing patient charts, input skills, and familiarity, but for those starting out there is no choice. It is important to find a system which is appropriate for your specialty, and which meets federal government requirements. Be aware that many broad-based systems may not be suitable for your specific needs. Sharing of medical information will be enhanced by the utilization of electronic medical records. Your system must be integrated with other systems within the hospitals you utilize, in your multi-specialty group, and ideally with other physicians with whom you consult. Another obvious advantage of electronic records will be legibility, as physicians are notorious for poor handwriting. Further, such patient information will be easily transmitted to other physicians outside your system when appropriate.

The physician and other health care provider must be able to pay attention to their patient even as they type away on their computers. A great deal of information is lost when attention is paid to the computer screen, rather than to the patient, where it is important to observe body language, the patient's eyes and the way he or she responds to your questions. I recently observed a nurse doing an emergency room patient intake facing her computer and asking questions of the patient who was on a bed behind her. She barely ever turned to look at the patient during the entire intake. I have had patients unhappily tell me that some doctors they had seen stared at their computers while asking questions and typing away but never looked at them during the whole time their history was taken. Health care providers must be trained to use their computers while talking to and looking at their patient. If they cannot, it might be more appropriate to input the information after the history is taken, or even after the patient has left the room.

Inputting must be done carefully. It is easy to make mistakes by hitting the wrong key. Such errors may be perpetuated in the system unless they are recognized. It is also easy to do a lot of box checking for items you may not have actually asked about, as for example in a long review of systems. Plaintiff attorneys will be looking for those type of input errors.

Integration with other physicians, hospitals, partners within a group, labs, radiology units, and pharmacies is obviously the great advantage of electronic medical systems. One will know immediately what care the patient has received from other physicians, what lab work and other studies have been done, what medications have been prescribed, and patient allergies. There will be pop-ups about possible drug interactions and potential allergic reactions. This information will be instantly available. Additionally, computers are able to search for information and can make it rapidly available.

Patients will appreciate the thoroughness of the electronic system, knowing all their medical information will be easily accessed by whatever physician or medical institution with which they may become involved. Over time, patients may be the beneficiaries of a computer flash drive containing their medical information which they would be able to carry with them. This technology is presently available on a limited scale provided by individual concierge physicians.

An issue of concern is that doctor-think and computer-think are not the same. Most computer models have been developed for billing and financial reasons. Their templates are not designed to work like physicians think. By using these templates, physicians are forced to model their thought processes to be like computers.

One of the big difficulties with electronic records is repetition. I often receive numerous pages of duplicate information when I receive records from those physicians or institutions which utilize electronic records.

Another issue could be the purity of the chart. By that I mean it is crucial that the information in the chart pertains only to the patient in question. It is possible for information from charts to be intermingled. I have been told by medical personal that charts have been received with information about another patient embedded in the requested information.

I also often receive complete charts when I requested only specific information. An inappropriate side effect of this situation is that information about highly personal medical issues – such as those related to sexual conditions, alcoholism, other addictions, or psychiatric illness which may be in the chart – become available for viewing by anyone who has access to the medical record. Electronic records are available to a great number of persons including physicians, nurses, ancillary medical personnel, and insurance company personnel who might be auditing the chart. Such chart viewers might have the need to see certain parts of the chart relating to their particular area of interest, but they should not necessarily be able to view the entire chart, which may contain sensitive personal information that might prove embarrassing to the person whose chart they are reviewing. This would be even more of an issue if the patient happened to be a fellow worker or someone with whom the viewer has a personal relationship.

Electronic medical records open up a whole new area of potential medical malpractice problems. Standard templates may encourage charting for services which were not performed. It is easy to click on multiple boxes just to get through the charting without actually asking the questions relating to what was checked. Templates should be individualized. Operative notes may be general and not specific to exactly what was done in the operating room. Notes may be signed without actually having been read. Inaccuracies may be missed. The same information may be repeated over and over. If there is an unrealized error, this error will be perpetuated throughout the chart. What is in the electronic chart is assumed to be accurate. Such may not be the case. An electronic trail is easy to follow. You can tell when the information was created, including time and date. You can tell who accessed the information and when. Alterations can be uncovered. Destroyed evidence can also be recovered. If there is evidence that information has been destroyed, courts can presume "spoliation," which means there is a legal assumption of wrongdoing by the party who destroyed the information. Any changes made to the record must be carefully noted as to what was changed, by whom, and when. Physicians must exercise great care when utilizing computerized medical records so as not to open themselves up to unexpected legal entanglements.

Computerization of your office will also be necessary for you to be able to participate in evidence-based medicine, which will become more and more important in medical decision-making. It is likely that reimbursement in the future will be determined by the usage of evidence-based medical care.

20

Coverage

You will need good on-call doctors for times when you may unavailable. Ideally these physicians will be as qualified and conscientious as you would be in providing prompt and appropriate responses to your patients' needs. Hopefully they will be as nice to your patients as you are. Situations will arise when the patient prefers you to the physician for whom you are covering, and will ask if they may switch to your practice. Your answer should be no. You do not want to be seen as soliciting patients from members of your on-call group.

A good answering service is a necessity. They should be prompt in response to calls, pleasant to your patients, and persistent in attempting to reach you or your on-call physician.

Applications for state licenses, hospital staffs, Medicare, Medicaid, and private insurance companies should be completed as soon as you know where you will be. This includes the various identity numbers needed. These can take weeks to many months to be approved.

21

Office Set-Up

If you are opening your own office, you will need equipment, furniture, and supplies.

Medical equipment will, of necessity, relate to your type of practice. You will need to decide how many rooms you will work in, and list what specific equipment will be needed in each type of exam room, lab, or minor surgery room. You will need to decide between leasing or buying, and whether extended warranties are worth their cost. Professional installation and training of your staff will be necessary for the more sophisticated equipment.

The staff offices will require desks, chairs, computers, phones, copiers, fax machines, postage machines, cabinets, storage areas, bookcases, and the like. Ditto for the medical staff offices.

The waiting room has to be furnished with comfortable seating, magazine racks or holders containing a variety of interesting, current, up to date reading materials, and coat racks. If you have enough space, it might be helpful to have a television on the wall with video information about your practice, or medically appropriate topics. Some patients also like to watch local programs while waiting, but be careful, as many patients are annoyed by the constant television chatter. Don't forget to allow seating in exam rooms for family members.

Chairs must be comfortable, sturdy, and have arms. Do not use couches or loveseats; patients don't like to sit next to strangers or other sick people in your waiting room without separation. Older patients, heavy patients, and pregnant patients need strong chairs with arms to allow themselves to be supported getting in and out of their seat. In my first office I purchased beautiful, comfortable, colorful, low to the ground designer chairs which looked beautiful but were very difficult for patients to get in and out of. Many patients, especially the pregnant and the heavy, found themselves rolling out of the chair onto the waiting room floor, and then hoisting themselves up. Funny to watch, embarrassing to the patients, horrifying to me. These chairs were quickly gone, to be replaced by appropriate sturdy chairs with arms.

A staff eating area may need a refrigerator, microwave, toaster oven, coffee maker, hot and cold water dispenser, sink, table and chairs, plates, cups, eating utensils, cleaning supplies, soap, and a vacuum cleaner.

You'll have to decide if you will need an in-office lavatory. That will be in part determined by your specialty: necessary for primary care, ob/gyn, urology, but not as important for those such as ophthalmology.

22

Summary

While I was a resident I took care of an elderly lady who was blind due to glaucoma, despite many years of clinic visits, and numerous doctor appointments. Every doctor who saw the lady over a ten year period mentioned in the chart that she had obtained whatever glaucoma medications which had been ordered for her. I apparently was the first physician who asked her if she had ever used the medications. When I asked to see her medications, she brought in a suitcase full of purchased but unopened eye drops dating back for over ten years. She had let herself go blind on purpose! After further investigation it turned out she lived alone, had been estranged from her daughter, and felt the only way she could get her daughter to take care of her was to create this disability. She was referred for psychiatric follow-up and care.

In the early years of my practice I ran a monthly eye clinic in Leadville a small mountain town. One day an elderly man was brought in by a concerned neighbor. The patient was legally blind due to cataracts, lived alone in a small cabin, was still driving, and while cooking would often set things on fire due his poor vision, causing great concern among his neighbors. I removed the cataract in one eye. The patient achieved 20/20 vision, resumed driving safely, and no longer set fires in his house. When I asked when he wanted to have the second eye operated on, his reply was, "I'm so happy to see with one eye I don't want to waste even one day of my life going through another operation." He never did have the second eye operated on, and lived happily without incident until his death years later.

In summary, medicine is a customer service business. We must relate to people in ways we would like to be treated ourselves. We must be available, accessible, and communicative. We must listen and explain in understandable terms. We must never be condescending or take things for granted. We are dealing with people's health. We must look and act like professionals, as should our staff. Our work environment should be clean, comfortable, and inviting. Our offices must be pleasant places for our patients to visit and for us to work. We must care and mean it. We must be passionate about our work. We are uniquely privileged to be privy to people's inner feelings, fears, and hopes. We often know more about our patients than anyone else, and should never abuse that trust. We have the opportunity to improve lives, often in unexpected ways. We are lucky and honored to be physicians.

Part V

The Future of Medicine

23

Thoughts for the Future

I diagnosed glaucoma in a highly educated, (Ph.D.), intelligent patient who refused to accept the diagnosis and refused to take his therapeutic eye drops. His peripheral vision began to deteriorate, so I recommended glaucoma surgery which he accepted despite his belief that he did not have glaucoma, and which was performed with good control of his intraocular pressure. He subsequently told his internist, who had referred the patient to me, that I would not treat his glaucoma! The internist laughingly told me not to worry, the patient complained to others that he, the internist, refuses to treat his hypertension.

What does the future hold for the practice of medicine? Huge change is on the horizon. Here are some of my predictions.

There will be a large influx of patients into the system while the number of physicians decreases, especially in primary care. Many physicians will retire earlier than originally planned, as reimbursements decrease, practice expenses continue to rise, and workloads increase. For senior physicians, job satisfaction and morale are diminishing as unreasonable demands from patients, insurance companies, and the government become the norm. They see the practice of medicine becoming a job, rather than a profession. When they retire early, not only does the system lose physicians, but the younger doctors lose valuable mentoring. Fewer medical students will choose primary care due to poor reimbursements and larger patient loads. Many doctors graduate with significant financial debts, often in the hundreds of thousands of dollars, and they see no hope of earning enough money in primary care to even begin to pay off their debt, let alone to be able to support a family. As a result of poor reimbursement, which will continue to worsen, physicians will opt out of Medicare and Medicaid in increasing numbers, making it more difficult for those patients to find a doctor. States will retaliate by insisting on mandatory participation in these programs in order to obtain licensing.

There will be minimal opportunity for young doctors to open their own offices, especially in urban areas. Most new physicians will join established groups, modeled after systems such as Kaiser, The Mayo Clinic, The Cleveland Clinic, The Henry Ford Health System, The MD Anderson Cancer Center, or other such groups around the country. Those doctors interested in academic medicine will become members of medical school staffs. Medical schools, which have traditionally been centralized centers for tertiary care referrals, will find themselves competing with private practitioners and groups in the marketplace by opening clinics for primary care and various specialties in outlying areas which would feed patients into the academic system. There will be an increase in multi-specialty groups, such as Precedent Health Partners developed in Denver, several years ago, which attempted to create a unique multi-specialty model, but failed as it was ahead of its time. One of the unusual features of Precedent was the concept of rewarding primary care physicians from the specialist income pool, thus acknowledging the importance to the specialists of the primary care referral base and helping compensate primary care physicians for their lower reimbursements. Single-specialty groups or organizations of same specialty physicians in one location, such as The Urology Center of Colorado, where a number of urologists banded together to build and equip a building unique for the practice of urology, will be formed. There also may be surgical centers of excellence created and staffed by physicians who basically provide only surgical services referred in by non-surgical physicians.

There will still be a place for solo physician or small practices in rural areas, but it is difficult to make such isolated practices attractive to doctors. Physicians like being able to discuss cases with other doctors. There are also issues of free time, vacations, burnout, on-call coverage, and continuing education for those who practice in isolated locations. Telemedicine will become more important, allowing rural physicians access to specialists. Face-to-face video consulting, along with the long distance reading of X-rays and MRIs, are programs already in use and which will grow in significance, especially for the care of patients with limited access to physicians. Rural outreach programs, where specialists fly in for consults and teaching, will be helpful. Foreign medical graduates will fill many rural medical needs.

In order to compensate for reduced reimbursement, physicians will become volume oriented. The result will be "zoom-care." Doctors will zoom in and zoom out of patient encounters, since reimbursement will be based on quantity, not quality.

Primary care will be provided by physician extenders, physician assistants, child health associates, nurses, midwives, and a variety of technicians. It is likely that a small number of primary care physicians will be responsible for a number of physician extenders in a practice. This will also be true for many specialties, such as ophthalmology, where optometrists and ophthalmic technicians will provide primary eye care. There will also be more foreign trained physicians assuming primary care responsibilities. Anesthesia is a problem in rural areas. Nurse anesthesia is more available than MD anesthesia, but that raises the question of responsibility and supervision. Is the surgeon, who may not know much about anesthesia, in charge in the OR, or is the nurse providing anesthesia responsible for his or her actions?

In many situations, especially group models, physicians will be salaried, rather than being paid based on productivity, as most are now. There will probably be a base salary together with some kind of incentive-based bonus structure over the base salary, which would encourage doctors to go the extra mile.

There will be an increase in the growth of concierge and boutique practices for those patients who can afford them, and for those physicians who have the appropriate practice demographic to provide such services.

Doctors in self-pay specialties, such as plastic surgery, will continue to do well, but will face stiffer competition as more doctors see the advantages of such specialties.

Physicians will be tempted to provide self-pay services outside their specialties, and some will prescribe medications or cosmetics for a fee. There will be an increase in internet prescribing for money, based on unsubstantiated medical information provided to a doctor who may have no relation to the patient requesting the medication.

THOUGHTS FOR THE FUTURE

Physicians who partner in ambulatory surgical centers will find such investments helpful in supplementing income, especially since they may find they earn more from the ambulatory center than from what they are paid for doing the surgery itself. One surgeon told me his surgery was a loss leader, as his reimbursement from the use of his ambulatory surgery center was greater than his surgical reimbursement. Hospitals will find themselves in partnership with doctors in such centers, or they stand to lose the most lucrative cases.

Hospitals will lobby to prevent the creation of physician-owned specialty hospitals.

24

Health Care System

Private health insurers will not stand idly by while the federal government mandates major changes in health care for the country. As the insurers lose the ability to refuse coverage to those most in need, they will develop other ways to create income. Co-pays will continue to increase, especially for visits to specialists. Deductibles will increase. Patients will be forced to come up with more and more money up front in order to receive medical care. Health insurance as we know it will become more like major medical insurance. First dollar coverage will be prohibitive, if it will even be available. The result will be that patients will be less likely to present for preventative care except where coverage is mandated by law. Due to up-front costs, patients will delay visits to physicians. They will thus be sicker before seeing their physicians, which will increase the significance of their problems which will then require more costly care than if they had presented earlier. There will be increased utilization of emergency rooms, putting greater burdens on hospitals.

The health care system as we know it must change dramatically.

The new system must provide efficient, high-quality health care in a cost efficient way for all. It should not be possible for a patient to be refused health insurance because of a pre-existing condition, or to have insurance canceled due to a serious medical condition. Lifetime caps should be removed. Insured medical care should be available for those below the poverty line who cannot afford to purchase insurance on their own. Private insurance companies exist to make money for their stockholders and their employees, not for the good of the insured or the providers of medical care. Their culture attempts to insure those who are healthiest, and to deny coverage to those who need care the most. Insurers negotiate the lowest payments for health care providers and hospitals, often forcing hospitals into bidding wars for contracts. These philosophies are unacceptable. Perhaps one answer might be to extend Medicare to all, so that everyone would be guaranteed quality basic medical care. Premiums would be based on a sliding income scale. Patients who could not afford the premiums would be subsidized by their state governments with help from the federal coffers. Those who wish to go beyond Medicare would be able to purchase extra or luxury insurance through private insurers. This would be the niche for private insurance companies. Such a two-tiered system would function for everyone's benefit. Basic care would be provided for all; those who could afford to purchase more sophisticated, more personal care should be allowed to do so.

Medicare fraud and abuse must be curtailed and if possible, eliminated. It must be understood, however, that honest unintentional errors by physicians' offices in coding and billing do not necessarily constitute fraud.

Pharmaceutical and medical device companies will fall under

increasing government restrictions and controls. Relationships between physicians and pharmaceutical companies will be tightly monitored. Physicians often do research with drug companies and give talks on behalf of these same companies. They are paid well for these endeavors. However, this does not necessarily mean that the doctor will skew his or her results for the advantage of the company, or encourage the use of certain pharmaceuticals inappropriately. It also should be understood that listening physicians can analyze the information provided and decide for themselves as to its value for their patients. As restrictions increase, and funding decreases, more and more innovative research and development will relocate outside the United States.

Patients will opt for less traditional alternative forms of health care. The internet will become ever more important as a source of advice and suggestions for self-care. Wellness programs provided by employers will offer advice on healthy lifestyles. Usage of supplements, herbs, and home remedies will increase. Acupuncture, homeopathy, and chiropractic remedies will become more popular. One of the advantages provided by practitioners in these programs is that they offer more personal attention to patients, which may be more beneficial than the treatments themselves, and which may make them less likely to be sued for malpractice.

25

Cost Containment

For many years I took care of a patient who had been deaf since birth and had Medicaid insurance. Her visits to the office were long and tedious, as all communication was through sign. Medicaid reimbursement was paltry, but at least the sign person she would bring was from an agency which billed Medicaid. After the American Disabilities Act was passed, everything changed. Now I was responsible for providing the sign person, so the agency billed me for their services. Their fee was far more than I received from Medicaid for seeing the patient. From then on, it cost me money every time the patient came in for an exam.

Cost containment will be a major concern in all areas of health care. Rationing health care dollars will be necessary. State governments will be more restrictive with regard to Medicaid availability. Eligibility will become more limited. Allowed procedures will be reduced. Age- related restrictions with regard to expensive procedures such as transplants, heart operations, artificial joints, and dialysis will be instituted in both Medicare and Medicaid. It will be important that good judgment be utilized in making such decisions. Age alone should not be the criteria. The general health and mental status of the patient are important. Some older patients are better suited to have sophisticated procedures than those who are younger. I know of a patient in his eighties who was automatically rejected for a kidney transplant at two institutions because he was over sixty-five, despite the fact he was in good health other than his renal status. He was able to procure a live donor, finally underwent a renal transplant at a third hospital, and is back to a happy healthy life off dialysis.

Perhaps funding could be based on a combination of government and patient cost sharing. Balance billing should be allowed. It seems unfair and unreasonable to prevent patients from spending their own money to improve the quality of their medical needs if they wish to do so and and are able to.

Major changes will be made in the way we provide end of life care as huge amounts of time and money are spent on expensive tests and treatments in often futile and inappropriate attempts to prolong life, both in those patients with terminal illnesses, and in the aged.

Cost for health care at the other end of the life spectrum, premature newborns, must also be examined. We expend major financial medical resources on tiny premature babies, many of whom have little hope of living normal functional lives. We have superb technology and highly skilled neonatologists and are thus able to prolong the lives of tiny babies who would not otherwise have survived. But where do you draw the line? This is an area fraught with social, political, and emotional issues which will not be resolved, yet will be a great financial drain on the health care system.

Research money will be more difficult to obtain. This will mean a greater percentage of available money will go to established laboratories, and to known researchers. Less money will be available for younger up and coming scientists, which will curtail creativity and reduce the pool of younger researchers. Since most research money is funded by the federal government, more scientists will turn to the private sector for funding.

Preventive health care, proper nutrition and exercise, together with tobacco, alcohol, and drug abuse control will be emphasized and rewarded as a way of reducing future health issues.

A new paradigm will need to be created with regard to physician work time, and hospital usage. New efficiencies will be created by the use of Saturday and Sunday office hours for physicians, and better utilization of hospital time on those days also. Weekends are underutilized both by physicians and by hospitals, while fixed expenses remain unchanged.

Many hospitals will close. In the present situation, hospitals are facing huge loses and high debts. Reimbursements often do not cover costs, and the number of uninsured patients is increasing. Decreasing revenues, decreasing reimbursements, and higher costs will lead to hospitals in great financial trouble, especially in big cities with low-income populations. As more hospitals close, the patient care burden will shift to the existing hospitals, putting pressure on their financial position. Reforms will be needed in the way hospitals operate, and the way they are reimbursed by both the state and federal governments, and by the private insurance companies.

26

Computers

Computers will have a dramatic effect on the practice of medicine. Personal care will be replaced by computer care. Physicians will find themselves utilizing automation in all aspects of medical care: collecting data, image gathering, recording findings, and making diagnoses. Decision-making for diagnoses and treatments will be determined to a great degree by evidence-based medical programs. Electronic medical records will become the norm. It will be crucial to provide safeguards for the information contained in electronic medical records. The risk of identity theft is real, and potentially devastating. Physicians will spend less time looking at and talking with patients, and more time looking at their computers. Physicians must protect against this. Initiative will be stifled. Physicians will follow computer recommendations.

27

Tort Reform

A lady came in for an eye exam and mentioned she had recently undergone eyelid surgery. I advised her the surgery had been done well and she had an excellent result. She began to cry. When I asked why she was crying, she pointed to a tiny wrinkle on the skin near her lids and said, "I'm very disappointed. I didn't have this wrinkle before the surgery."

Tort reform will need to be instituted across the country, not just in a few states such as Colorado. Ideally, medical courts would be established, and staffed by judges with medical expertise, together with panels of physician jurors, rather than by juries selected from the population as a whole. Medical cases are far too complicated and emotionally charged to be understood by lay persons. Participating attorneys should also have medical expertise and should be paid reasonably but not outrageously for their services. Fair and reasonable award standards should be set. Awarded monies should flow directly to the appropriate patient, or their guardians.

28

House Staff Training

As a medical intern at Boston City Hospital I had many never to be forgotten experiences.

One night after midnight, following a particularly long grueling day, I was headed for bed when I passed a fellow intern working on an extremely ill patient. I stopped to help, and after several hours and a lot of effort we stabilized the patient. I was then able to get to bed for a few hours; the patient did well and was eventually discharged. It turns out he owned a Chinese restaurant in Boston, and a few days after his discharge he and his family brought in homemade Chinese food for us all to share. A nice treat for the doctors and nurses, and a nice example of the comradeship which develops when house-staff members help each other.

It was dark, long after midnight. The ward was quiet, the patients were asleep and I was alone in the interns' and residents' office finishing my charts for the night. I heard a sound, looked up, and saw a creepy man in the doorway. He had a strange look on his face. His hand was in his overcoat pocket as if he were holding a gun. He stared at me. I stared back, incredulous. I had no idea who he was or how he got there, but we were alone and he acted as though he wanted to shoot somebody. Everything felt surreal. For an instant I thought I was dreaming. He walked into the room still staring at me, his hand still in his pocket. After the initial shock passed, I felt I'd better try to talk to disarm him. He came closer. I got up, still talking quietly, and decided my only chance would be to get close enough to jump him before he could shoot. I kept talking and moved slowly toward him. It worked! I was able to grab and hold him down while pulling his arm out of his coat. There was no gun! Instant relief. Security took him away. I never saw him again. I didn't finish any more charts that night.

My first child was born during the second month of my internship. My wife went into labor; I was tied up with sick patients and was unable to get out to go home to drive her to the hospital. She was to deliver at Massachusetts Memorial Hospital, not far from Boston City Hospital. She ended up driving herself while in labor to my hospital where I was able to meet her for the rest of the trip to where she was to deliver.

One weekend during internship, my parents came up from New York to see the baby and to visit us for the weekend. I had just finished a stint where I had been up working for three days and two nights with minimal sleep. I remember sitting down on the bed to change clothes and waking up twenty-four hours later. My wife entertained my parents, took care of the baby, and by the time I awakened, they had gone back to New York.

One night a huge man was admitted to our ward from the emergency room. He was as big and as strong as a professional football lineman. He was lying asleep on the gurney but as he arrived on the floor he suddenly awakened and became violent. He grabbed the strap from the gurney and swung it around with great force, with the buckle end out, thus creating a dangerous weapon and making it impossible for anyone to get near him. Finally after a lot of ducking and dodging, several large orderlies and I were able to hold his arms long enough for the nurse to inject a sedative, which took hold after a while and ended the danger.

One day I was working upstairs on the ward when I heard gunshots. I looked out the window and saw lots of people running around in the vicinity of the emergency room. It turned out a gang member had been shot in a fight. He was brought to the Boston City Hospital emergency room. The shooter and his gang members came to finish him off, and got into a shoot out with members of the injured man's gang. The Boston police were called and quickly ended the disturbance. Lots of gurneys were overturned and lots of glass was broken, but happily the flying bullets injured no one.

Under the rules of the Accreditation Council for Graduate Medical Education (ACGME), those in resident training today have been taught to restrict their hours, and have lost the incentive to do as much as they can to learn as much as they can. These policies are an attempt to change the previous intern and residency programs in which doctors in training worked long hours, often with little or no sleep, in order to take care of their patients, cover the wards and the emergency rooms, attend conferences, present patients to staff members on rounds, follow up on lab work, write up charts, read journals, and do whatever mundane work needed to be done during their time on service. Physicians in training were exhausted and sleep deprived and always under the gun, expected to be available at all times for their patients, their senior residents, and their attending physicians. Patient care was often compromised by doctor fatigue. However, patients overall did well, and we, the house staff, learned a great deal. We also developed comradeship, a sense of working together, pride, and accomplishment. We made it through the system; so should the next group. We developed a sense of obligation to be there for our patients, and for each other, no matter what, no matter when, and no matter how late. When you take care of sick patients, all days and nights are the same.

There is a need for change in this teaching model, but the ACGME has swung the pendulum too far. House staff does need more rest in order to provide optimal patient care. However, they also need to take care of patients, and attend conferences, lectures, and surgical procedures in order to learn, and should not be totally restricted by a timecard, which can be used as an excuse to refuse to attend an important learning experience. I have talked to several residency program directors who have expressed frustration at the unwillingness of house staff to go beyond their allotted hours in order to see an interesting patient, attend an important lecture, or scrub in on an unusual surgical case. These young doctors are the ones who will be out there in the future making important decisions about patient care. They are intelligent and responsible, and should be treated as such. How else will they learn to function adequately when they enter the real world and assume patient responsibility? The ACGME must allow flexibility in resident training hours, so as to allow doctors in training to make their own decisions as to how their time should be spent. They need to learn how to manage their time wisely, and how to prioritize their activities. They must learn how to make choices. If they don't learn it now, when will they?

29

Quality of Life

There will be major changes in quality of life issues for new physicians. They will have to be able to balance their personal and professional lives in a way which will be far different from previous generations of physicians. They will be willing to give up some level of income and autonomy in order to work fewer hours and have more family and non-work time.

Over all, physicians of the future will have better quality of life, work fewer hours, feel less responsible to their patients, have less incentive to be there for their patients, feel less obligated to work long hours and to stay late, and will probably make less money. A majority of physicians will be salaried. They will be more likely to pass after-hours patients on to emergency rooms or on-call physicians rather than staying to see them personally. They will look at being a doctor as a job, with standard hours like everyone else — coffee breaks, lunch hours, and a regular schedule. There will be increased government and insurance company oversight and control. There will be less individual autonomy and more decision-making by computer. This is a new culture for physicians, perhaps better for quality of life issues, but not necessarily better for patient care and the pride of being a physician, a member of an incredibly wonderful profession.

30

Hope for the Future

During my career I have had many interesting and rewarding patient experiences. I have shared a few stories in these pages. The vast majority of my patients have been appreciative, and it has been a pleasure to have helped make their lives better. I have received hundreds of gifts and letters of thanks, all of which have vindicated my choice of becoming a physician. I wish the same sense of fulfillment and happiness for all those of you who choose to follow the same path. There is nothing like the joy of the practice of medicine!

The future of medicine is in your hands. You are the doctor. Don't lose sight of why you wanted to be a doctor and why you worked so hard to get where you are. You will be working in a culture of government and insurance company control. Decisions will be computer driven, but you will have the ability to override the computer, to make your own decisions. You, the physician, have the right, the credentials, the training and the intelligence to make choices. Remember when you are in a room with a patient it's you and the patient, one on one. Physicians are looked at in a special way by their patients. People let us into their lives in a way that is not available to any other person. Always recognize you are a physician, not "a provider"; your patient is a person, not "a book of business." You will be expected by the patient to make decisions which are best for him or her, not necessarily best for the government or the insurance company. Never forget that however rich or poor, famous or unknown, powerful or meek, the person is front of you is equally worried about his or her medical condition. We are healers. We are allowed to make choices that affect the lives of all we care for. We are privileged to be physicians. Control is in our hands to do right for our patients, despite the external forces under which we operate. Medicine is a joyful profession, and it is a profession, not just a job. It is an honor to be a physician, to be trusted above all others. We can all be proud to be called "Doctor."

CPSIA information can be obtained at www.ICGtesting.com

224919LV00002B/2/P

9 781432 770501